F CANCER

A FIGHTING MINDSET TO GET THROUGH CANCER

KENTE HARRIS

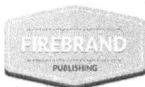

FIREBRAND
PUBLISHING

Firebrand Publishing publishes in a variety of print and
electronic formats and by print-on-demand. For more
information about Firebrand Publishing products,
visit https://firebrandpublishing.com
ISBN: 978-1-941907-64-1 paperback
ISBN: 978-1-941907-58-0 eBook
Printed in the United States of America

CONTENTS

F*ck Cancer   1
Questions   15
Chemo   21
Does The Whole World Have
Cancer?   27
Why Me?   33
After   39

ABOUT F CANCER

This is a vigorous, powerful story of one man's tireless effort to not only survive a cancer diagnosis and treatment, but to increase his strength and resolve and emerge victorious!!!

In sharing his mindset and experiences in this book, Kente truly hopes to help others in their search for strength and direction. Whatever life challenge come your way, take solace from this powerful and personal experience.

F*CK CANCER

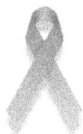

W hat the fuck!
   Never in my wildest dreams did
I think that turning 40 meant I would be
looking cancer in the face. Having been a
single dad at the age of 18 to 20, and raising
two kids totally on my own, I figured by the
time they grew up I would get my life back.
That's why I started having kids so early.

I had my first kid at 18 years of age, and
the next at 20. I thought by doing so, I would
be finished with raising kids at a very young
age. There I was at 39 years old, jumping for
joy because I was finally coming to the end of
raising kids. One was now 20 and the other
was turning 18, so yes, I was so looking forward to my 40th birthday because this would

mean *Freedom*! Time to enjoy my life alone. But little did I know, cancer was lurking around the corner.

It was late September 2017. I was on a small vacation for the weekend in St Louis with my 89 year old client. It was a special treat from me to him. After all, he became my cool little friend, even though he was my client. I thought of him as a grandfather I'd never had. I always wanted to have a grandfather I could go on vacation with.

My job was to take care of the elderly, somehow, I always ended up with the old man. I figured this was my opportunity for my grandfather void to be filled. The funny thing is, even though my client was a millionaire, I did not want any of his money to pay for this boys road trip. I figured, since his wife was off on vacation in Florida with my mom, I needed to do something with just the two of us, so off to St Louis we went.

During the trip, my head started hurting. The pain was so bad, I went to the store and bought Excedrin maximum strength pills for my horrible headache. I took two tablets. An hour and half passed, and my head was still hurting the same. So I took two more tablets. Another hour passed and still no change.

Recalling my training as a medication technician, and knowing how dosages are administered, I knew something was wrong. There had to be a much bigger problem because I continued to have constant pain with the large doses of headache medicine I took.

If I'm taking pain meds, and the pain is not relieved, or making any changes over a four-hour span, I know something else must be wrong. Suddenly, I also felt a lump on the left side of my neck. This pain was now shooting from this lump to the entire left side of my head with no letting up. No matter how much pain meds I took over the weekend vacation, nothing helped to relieve or even affect the pain.

As soon as I got back home, I made a doctors appointment knowing it would take a while to get in. On the day of the doctors visit, I was referred directly to ENT, the Ear Nose and Throat specialist. The wait for that appointment also took a long time.

On the day of the ENT visit, I was told I needed to do a biopsy.

What is a biopsy? I had no idea what it was. I was told that I could watch on the tv screen while they stick a needle in the lump on the side of my neck. I asked the specialist why were they going to stick a needle in my neck. She told me they will extract fluids to send off to pathology, or testing.

Then, I was told I would have to wait for the results. The wait felt like an eternity to say the least.

The day I went in to hear the results the ENT specialist delivered the news. He said, "You have nasopharyngeal cancer ."

I didn't act shocked or surprised. To be honest, I kind of figured I had cancer, because the lump I felt in my neck, felt like the same lump I felt in my stepmom's breast 10 years earlier. She was diagnosed with breast cancer. So, I really wasn't that surprised.

That day, I went home and got on with my day as if I didn't hear something totally devastating. That's my personality. When I hear something bad, I never let it shake me. However, when the ENT doctor told me where the cancer in my sinus was located, I was taken aback. A few years earlier I developed a problem with my nasal passage. At the time, it was necessary for my primary doctor to prescribe a prescription nasal spray. I think the cancer started developing from that time.

My primary doctor apologized to me. She said that if steps were taken, to take a much closer look earlier, then she may have seen the cancer developing in my sinus cavity earlier.

Take this as a WARNING: If you notice any changes in your body, especially when you are a certain age, ask your doctor to investigate it. The fact that you are experiencing those new changes could mean there is something growing or forming.

Next, I was sent directly to oncology aka the cancer center. This is where I learned about my treatment plan. While the doctor was talking all, I heard was *blah blah blah blah blah* and *chemo, radiation*.

The ironic and crazy thing about this visit was that to my surprise, this was the same doctor who treated my stepmom for her breast cancer for over 13 years. My stepmom only had one daughter, my baby sister. I became the spokesperson for her during her final days.

I was the one who made all the decisions concerning her health. When she passed July of 2017, I was the one that had to bury her. You can do the math and see how many months it was, from July to September, when I was first diagnosed with cancer. Surely, one can't write such a story.

I was told that my treatment would have to be scheduled in two different locations, which I call, *poor people problem*. Chemo would be done by my stepmom's doctor and radiation would be done at a different location across town. When I met the radiation doctor, he began to talk about a treatment plan and the same thing happened to me. The only thing I left there remembering was, *blah blah blah blah* again. The only thing I do remember him saying was that I was going to lose thirty to forty pounds! I was already so skinny. It made them feel I might need a feeding tube. After I heard about the feeding tube, I heard nothing else!!! Just, *blah blah blah blah*. It was like I kept coming in and out of *blah blahness* lol.

When he was done talking, I told him that I wished doctors didn't tell people so much because that can make people go into what I call *cancer Depression*. I know it's his job to educate me as to what I am about to embark on and what to look forward to but it was scary.

He made a dentist appointment for me, because it is common practice for people who are about to embark on radiation therapy to treat nasopharyngeal cancer. This requires radiation to the head and neck.

He said that most people who go through this type of treatment tend to have really bad teeth problems causing excruciating pain, so he advises everyone to go see the dentist. That way if they have any bad teeth or teeth that needed to be pulled, they should be pulled before radiation begins. If you start treatment without fixing any problems, and your teeth start hurting, you can't get those teeth pulled until after treatment is over.

When I went to see the dentist, he did an x-ray of my entire mouth. Then he had the nerve to tell me that I needed to have all my *DAMN* teeth pulled out. He then sent me directly to oral surgery.

When I got upstairs to oral surgery, I told the oral surgeon, "I am just 40 years old and there is no way I am getting all my teeth pulled." The only way I would agree to get all my teeth pulled out was if they were going to give me implants the same day they pulled all my teeth. I told them that if they couldn't do that, then they're not pulling my teeth. I told them, that I'd walk, because I already knew from the beginning, that no one was going to dictate the outcome of me going through cancer treatment.

While all this was in motion, I was getting ready for a trip to Jamaica for my grandmother's 80th birthday party. I told the oncologist that I was not going to do any treatment until I return from Jamaica. You see, I was the organizer for my grandmother's birthday party and there was no way in hell I would have missed my grandma's 80th birthday party. Nothing was going to stop me, not even finding out I had cancer and that I needed to start treatment right away.

I began Chemo and Radiation two weeks after I returned from Jamaica. During the two weeks before treatment started, I went shopping for things I'll call *cancer preparation shopping*. I bought weight gaining supplements, supplements high in protein, and a big cup for larger amounts of water. When I got home from *cancer preparation shopping,* I put everything I bought on the counter in my kitchen. I stood back and looked at all this stuff, and thought to myself, *this SHIT looks like I am accepting this cancer as a part of my life.* At that moment I took everything I bought and tossed it in the trash and said, "FUCK NO! I am not going to make you be a part of my life."

From that day on I made the decision that I would never absorb cancer in my life. I told myself if it comes a point that I lose my hair, I would never wear those *accepting cancer hats!* The ones you see most people with cancer wearing on their bald heads. To me the ones that go out and purchase them caps, are the ones that are making and okaying cancer to be a part of their life. I would not bring anything for the cancer to my house. I did not want to bring anything that has to do with cancer in my house. It was my way of saying cancer will never be welcome in my house.

I told my sister about my cancer diagnosis. I told her only to tell my brother, sisters, and dad. I did not want my mom to know because I knew she would be so heart broken. I just wanted to do my treatment and get it over with, without her finding out, but little did I know she would find out anyway. I had forgotten that we both worked with the same client.

The day she found out, I know she cried all the way home, and it broke my heart. Finding out I had cancer didn't faze me, but the hurt it caused my mom, was devastating to me. I told her to cry only once and that's it. I told her and my siblings to never say a word to anyone about me having cancer. To me, I felt that when you find out you have cancer and you tell the world, the world will deem you sick or dead, when that is the least thing that should be on your mind. It's like they put energy into the universe about your faith, before you get a chance to put your fighting faith in the universe. That is why I chose not to tell anyone outside of my immediate family. I told my family, "We are only going to talk about it ONCE and that is it." I told them, "Don't call me every day asking me how I am doing, PERIOD."

That's why I didn't want the world to know I had cancer, because what people don't realize is that they are doing more harm when they ask someone with an illness, especially cancer, how they are doing and how they are feeling every day. The person that's going through the illness might not be feeling sick until someone starts asking, "How you doing, how you feeling?" If you know someone who is going through cancer and or cancer treatment, that doesn't mean you need to talk to them every day about it. They don't need the *cancer* sick concerns reminder, daily. Just try to treat that person as you would if you didn't know they had cancer. Unwittingly bringing it up constantly, you are constantly reminding that person of the first time they heard the word cancer.

My first day of chemo was like any other day to me. I had already decided that this problem needed to be fixed, and this was what was needed to be done. This is my personality. When there is a problem I never let it get me down. I live my life saying, "before I get sad about something that I am going though, I turn it into anger."

I don't get angry at others, but at what it is that's trying to make me sad. The anger in me brings out the strength in me. Don't misunderstand me, I knew that going through chemo and radiation therapy would not be a walk in the park. I knew and saw how both of them destroyed people's sprit and morale. I told myself to never let that negativity get a hold of me. I told myself from day one that no matter how hard it gets, I will keep my spirit positive. I willed *my sprit to never get down, no matter what.*

I asked my oncologist about the different kinds of chemo. I asked him which one is stronger, which one would make my hair fall out? I chose to go with the one with the smaller dosage with a longer treatment schedule, than the high dosage with a shorter treatment schedule.

My chemo treatment would be in one location, then I would have to drive 3 miles to the other location (*poor people problem*) for radiation. I did that everyday until my treatment was complete. I keep saying poor people problem because I imagine that if I had better health insurance, maybe I would have been referred to a cancer center that had radiation and chemo therapy, under the same roof. What wealthy person do you know that would have to drive to two different locations in order to get radiation and chemo therapy treatment? NONE OF THEM!

This urges me to keep saying *"poor people problem"*, because, as poor people we take what we can get. When we're trying to survive, we are used to this kind of treatment so much so, it becomes our norm.

QUESTIONS

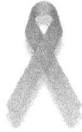

Questions about the different types of Chemo. I wanted to know what to expect with this treatment, and how will it affect me once it entered my body. This influenced my decision to ask a lot of questions. Even if you ask questions every day, my motto is, IF YOU THINK IT, ASK IT.

I had a lot of questions for my doctor to answer, and he did. I wanted to be sure that the person responsible for my treatment, for something that's so life threatening, is well educated on what needs to be done. Never think that just because they're a doctor, you must simply leave your life in their hands without asking questions, because at the end of the day you know your body the best.

The doctor knows how to give and prescribe medication, and have knowledgeable insight on the disease at hand. Remember it's your body, you tell it how to move, what mood you're going to be in, and how to think and feel. So, you and you alone can tell your body what's going in it and how it might make you feel and how you will react to those feelings. Let the doctor do his part. TRUST IN HIS KNOWLEDGE AS YOU TRUST IN YOUR BODY during this process.

One thing I asked the oncologist was, "if he was a teacher, would he be a teacher that just gave his students a lecture and then let them figure out everything that is needed for an exam without caring who passes or fails?

"Or would he be a teacher that would give a lecture, and also do whatever was necessary to make certain all his students understand the lecture?

"Would he care that all his student pass his exam?"

His answer to these questions would determine if I would let him be the oncologist to treat me. Understand, if he was going to be the teacher that doesn't care much whether his students pass or fail, then he certainly wouldn't care if his patients do well or not while undergoing chemo.

At the end of the day always remember, no matter what, you're always in control. That same day I went over to the radiation department aka, PETs Center. This is where I asked the same question. Both the oncologists gave me the answer I was looking for. Believe me, if any of them didn't give me answers that would make me feel comfortable, then they would be told exactly that, and I would have taken my *cancer ridden ass elsewhere,* lol.

When both doctors told me what both treatments would do to my body, I left both appointments and went to Whole Foods and bought, *Turkey mushroom tabs, vitamin c improve absorb ultra tabs, elderberry, graviola, vitamin d3 2000 IV.* Immediately, I began dumping them in my body every day, after I came home from work.

Oh yeah! I said "work."

I went to work every day throughout my entire treatment. The crazy thing is my client died on the last day of my treatments. I was with him when he took his last breath. When he passed, I left, and went to do my radiation and chemo. Then I came back and cleaned him up, and get him ready for the funeral home to pick him up. I then carried on with my day as if nothing happened.

I decided to purchase the supplements because I wanted to make sure that whatever chemo and radiation was going to destroy in my body, would be replaced immediately. No doctor was going to tell me differently.

As I previously said, you know your body best, better than any doctor. Always remember that doctors are only trained and educated to care for what's at hand. That same day I called my mom and told her that I wanted her to make soup. I love when my mom makes soup for me.

She is vegan, but her soup tastes so good I can't tell the difference between other soups with meat. I also asked my cousin to order me the fattiest pork she could get from the local Price Choppers. Then, I asked my sister to cook the pork for me. She knows how I like it.

Jerk Pork is my weakness, especially when it has a lot of fat on it. I also love *turkey tails* with collard greens.

I did this because I knew I had to give everything I had to fight this *bitch* called *cancer.* I remember the doctor said that radiation and chemo destroys cells, so I asked him what builds cells. I was told that protein builds cells. That's why I got the fattiest pork and turkey tails and my mom's soup. I came to the idea that if I dumped a lot of protein into my system, it could help to replace some of the damaged cells.

CHEMO

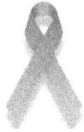

The first day I got that thing, *chemo* in my body, I didn't think of it as *I am doing chemo*, I thought of it as, *I am getting powers in my veins.*

I made sure I drank a lot of water because in my head I needed to flush that *shit* out my system as soon as possible. I wanted to get it out, so I drank lots and lots of water, so I would pee a lot. I'm not sure if that made any difference, but as I say, "It's your body, you know it better than any doctor, because that little bit of saline they give to you, doesn't seem like nearly enough fluid to me.

I thought, *I need to keep my kidneys and liver flushed, because I didn't want the build-up of chemo in my system making me weak.* No doctor was going to tell me otherwise. I wasn't even sad to go to the cancer Center/PETs Center. I actually looked forward to going each day because in my head, I was like, *let's go*! I mean, why be sad about going, as if that was going to make the cancer just up and disappear. Mostly, it helped to not think about being there.

At the cancer center, I made so many jokes, that a lady next door came over and said her husband was over there cracking up at what I was saying. She thanked me for making them laugh. She wanted to thank me for making her husband laugh, because he was having a down day. If you know my personality, you would know that by the end of my chemo treatment, everyone in that cancer section knew who I was. I make fun out of everything. I could be dying and know that I am, and I would still make fun about dying. I mean, why be sad? If it's out of your hands, just be happy. That's what I choose to do. If that situation presents itself.

At the center, I complained. I started complaining about the awful and dreadful music they play over the *damn* intercom. They call it calming music. I call it death music.

Like, who wants to sit here taking chemo treatment and listen to *"death music"* lol. I looked around at everyone strung up to their chemo machine, laying there looking like "corpses" lol.

I told my sister, if I could have it my way I would have everyone up and dancing while still strung up to those damn machines. It's like the patients come to the cancer center with an accepting, defeated spirit, just laying there waiting for whatever comes. Me being crazy, I told the doctor I want to be able to walk around with the machine. There was no way I was just going to lay there as if I was accepting cancer. I asked the doctor, "Do these people ask as much questions as I do?"

He said, "No".

I said, "So they just come here, sit and take whatever you give to them with not much question?" I told him, "Well not me! I need to know everything, as should everyone who embarks on such journey".

One thing I would encourage everyone is to find your where your strength is. When you do, put yourself in that mind frame. Don't come out of that frame of mind until your treatment is over. For me, I put my myself in the frame of mind as if I am a wounded dragon, staying still until it's time for me to rise and breathe the fire. It is like playing sick and wounded, but still having the strength to fight if need be. That's where I put my mind throughout my treatments. Take one day to cry, after that, no more crying. *There is no crying in strength.* Don't ask the question, Why me? It will never be answered, so spare yourself the headache.

When you leave treatment, never go home to lay in bed or lounge around like a wounded or sick animal. Go out, take the kids, husband, wife, or dog out. Continue your day as if you're not a bit phased by this bitch (cancer).

Yes, I'm saying bitch because every morning I wake up to brush my teeth and wash my face I always look in the mirror and say, "Bitch I know you've come for me but, fuck you."

I said this every morning before I went to get my treatment. I said it with such force and strength. It's like I was telling cancer, "Let's fucking go to war, I am ready and not scared." I know these words might not be for kids or some adults, but for once, I will give myself the go ahead and use them, because I feel it can give others the strength to fight.

Remember that monster comes for anyone. If you need to get angry and it helps, do it with no explanations and no apologies. Going through something like this will take you to that place. I'd rather my readers yell and cuss, than cry and be sad about something they can't change.

The thoughts about cancer still lingers way after treatment, because every time you feel sick or have a pain in that same area, your mind goes, *what the hell is this now?* If and when that happens to you, try what I do and say, "Get the fuck out my thoughts". Then say to yourself, *they got it all and for that I am certain*, and move on. Don't ever let the fear of cancer ever return or haunt you for the rest of your life. Just go back to your normal life as if that bitch (cancer) didn't just try to come for you.

DOES THE WHOLE WORLD HAVE CANCER?

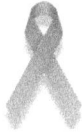

When that 5 years marker comes and you hear those words that you're officially clear of cancer, I want you to go back to that mirror. Stare yourself dead in the face and say again, "Bitch you came for me but fuck you." Say it with everything you got in you. This is to tell that bitch called cancer that you're not the one to mess with next time.

Maybe you might be one not to use foul language or let your kids use foul language, but in this case I say it's very fitting. Trust me, the God over Israel that I serve won't judge me for using such words, because even he has a sense of humor, and I believe any God you chose to serve won't judge you either.

Find something to lose yourself in, like your favorite TV show. Listen to your favorite artist, or try to watch things that will make you laugh. Laughing is good for you during this time. Simply find a hobby, or start working on a project you have been longing to start. Anything to keep your mind from letting the thoughts of that bitch (cancer) come in.

Find a group to belong to. Just make sure it is not a cancer group. Remember, you're just going through cancer, it is not a part of your life, so you don't need a group to keep reminding you of such a horrible time and challenge in your life.

I want you to go out and get yourself a new attitude. Change your hair color, get a new haircut, change your style of clothing. Show off that new you. I would say, if you were someone that never used to wear a certain type of clothing, start doing so. This might be surprising and come as a shock to your family members. Just do it for about three months with no apologies, and no regrets. To put it simply, do something out the box. Maybe there is something you've always wanted to do, but never had the courage to do. Beating cancer should give you all the courage you need.

FYI please, please, please don't take, or let anyone take any of those horrendous cancer pictures of you. You don't need that kind of reminder of such a depressing and painful time in your life. So, don't let anyone convince you that if you take these kind of pictures it will show you how far you have come. That's ludicrous!

Those memories should be buried and never to be spoken of ever again. Hearing the news that you're officially clear from cancer, is one way to free yourself forever. If there are no pictures, there will be no reminders or memories. It's like something I always tell the kids in my family, including my own. When they were at the age to start changing their teeth, I always told them never to smile in pictures once their teeth fell out because they will regret those pictures when they get older, especially when it is time to show off family photos to strangers. I always told them not to smile without teeth LOL. They don't need those type of memories. So why would anyone want the memories of battling that bitch called cancer that came for you?

The funny thing is, I never heard of the cancer I had, nasopharyngeal. Then, I found out that my best friend's sister was diagnosed with the same type of cancer that I had. She had finished her treatment years prior, then it returned in her brain. While my best friend was telling me this, she still didn't know anything about my diagnosis. Remember I said I didn't want anyone to know about me having cancer, only my family. As I mentioned earlier, I did not want anyone to put illness in the universe with my name on it. I believe that what you put in the universe will come back to you. I kept it a secret because I didn't want anyone to treat me as if I was sick, or have and show pity for me. That is not the route I chose to take. Not once did I ever let myself think that my faith would be the same as my best friend's sister.

At the time, a doctor my sister worked with was going through the same kind of cancer as well. She told me what it was doing to him. It wasn't good. He lost a lot of weight and his situation required an ENG tube inserted, to feed him. Yet, hearing all that bad news, never once made me worried, because I knew my mind was on whooping this bitch cancer's ass. So, I was ready to fight. The point is, just because you've heard that someone may have gone through the same kind of cancer you're going through, doesn't mean you and them carry the same faith. Just put in your mind that your fight is way, way, way different than theirs.

A couple of months later I saw my neighbor walking to his mailbox. He looked skinny. His shirt was open, and I noticed he had a trach, (tracheotomy) and a feeding tube. I asked him what was going on with him. He told me that he was going through cancer treatment too. I was like, "What the fuck. Is the whole world going through cancer treatment?" I told him if anyone could beat cancer I knew he would be the one, because he's a man of such inner and outer strength.

That was two years after my landlord wrote me to let me know he too was going through cancer treatment, both him and my neighbor. I understood why they had it. Both of them are chain smokers. The funny thing is, when I found out my neighbor had cancer, I felt kind of guilty because whenever he did any yard work for me, I always asked him if there's something I can get him. He would always tell me to get him a carton of his favorite cigarettes. So, in a way, I felt as though I had contributed to him having cancer. I can clearly see the reason why they both had cancer. This is where I say, "But why the hell did I get mines lol". Ask yourself that question, then say, "Fuck it," that way it won't haunt you to keep asking yourself questions. Just get that mind of yours in fighting mode.

WHY ME?

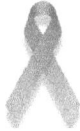

As far as those who are in favor of, pastors, priests, and nuns, I say keep them far away from you. They mean well, but what they don't understand is that every time they come by to ask if you need them to pray with you, they are contributing to your mind's defeat. They mean well, but I don't know who told them it was appropriate to pray for people going through any kind of life-threatening illness. Who wants to see them, when you are laying there receiving treatment. What they don't understand is, every time they visit, it makes people feel the severity of their illness, and that their life must be in really bad shape. People will feel that they must be at death's door. So, for all you religious messengers lol, please really think about it, before you come around asking people if you can pray for them, because you just might be making them feel like they have one foot in the grave.

One day I was receiving my treatment and a pastor came by my section and asked me if I needed prayer. I told his ass no, with a look like what the fuck! I wasn't trying to be rude, but that's the look I gave him. It was at that time I realized just how sick I was. I'd never seen myself as being sick before his ass showed up. Then he had the nerve to ask me if I believed in God. I said, "Yes I do." I told him I didn't want anyone to pray for me because I believe that God can hear me on his own, so I didn't need him to pray for me.

Sometimes when you are going through something life threatening, it is best for you to be careful who you permit to send God your prayer. Just because they call themselves Pastor, Priest, or Nun, it doesn't mean they have a better relationship with God, than you do. Be confident that your faith is strong enough to get through to your God. He will hear you, and take care of you.

Even though your appearance may change due to significant hair and weight loss, or discoloration of your skin due to radiation and chemo therapy, don't allow that to matter to you, because that's what cancer wants to do to you. It wants you to be down, depressed, and sad. This is where your strength will come in handy. When these appearance changes begin, look at yourself and say, "This is only for now, but as soon as my treatment is over, I know for sure what I am going to look like after this."

You can say, "cancer will never get me to the door of defeat." Look at yourself and say, "I already knew what was to come. In order for me to go to battle with you, I am going to wear my bald head, discolored skin and weight loss with proudness, because I already put in my mind that this was to come."

This is why I didn't tell anyone what I was going through because my mind was already made up with all the changes to come. You don't want to allow anyone to come in and try to take the strength you worked so hard to build, and turn it into pity. Pity to me is affirming or accepting the mind's weakness.

Going through such an ordeal showed me I had way more strength in me, maybe more than I realized. Yes, I ran marathons and did triathlon competitions, and I knew I had a strong mind, but never would I have thought all that would be tested. The funny thing is, I ran a 5k for scleroderma, October 2017. I came in third place that day. I thought we were just coming to run for a cause, but at the end they started giving out medals, and I found out I finished in third place. I was kind of upset because had I known there was going to be a medal ceremony after the race, I would have ran faster.

My competitive nature would driven me to really compete. They thought I was running for a cause, but little did they know I was running just to keep myself and my mind busy from thinking about cancer and my upcoming treatment. For me, going through cancer became like a fueling machine, because it only made me want to go after my dreams with increased energetic force. I feel unstoppable chasing my dreams.

One of my dreams was writing a book, but never in my wildest dreams did I ever think it would be about me having cancer and going through cancer treatment. But if I can empower the mind of a child, mother, father, aunt, uncle, niece, nephew, husband, or wife by sharing my story and my frame of mind while going through cancer and cancer treatment, then it was well worth me taking the time to write this book. The funny thing is I hate writing, but thanks to that bitch cancer, I was given the power of motivation to accomplish my goals and dreams, so going through cancer just might not be a bad thing after all.

Sometimes in life, God may put us through things to give us a push. God may use the things and tools he has blessed us with to accomplish our dreams. Maybe it's not simply for your goals and dreams. Maybe it's for you to be a better you, or for you to make amends with a loved one. Who knows, the question will remain out there. Try to understand what God is trying to tell you. For me I know it was my goals and dreams because he has blessed me with such a gift that I was not using. So, if you get diagnosed with cancer, don't just absorb it as a death sentence. Just get your mind in fighting mode as if you're going into battle, because in the end you will find that it will fuel you with such a force of energy to persue your goals and dreams. You might want to do things differently than you did before cancer. Your outlook on life may be affected and be different. It will make you feel like you want to take on the world, go on all the trips you've ever wanted to go on, and you will never want to put off any life outings, parties, birthdays, anniversaries, or special time with family, in fear that one day that dirty bitch cancer just might show back up, but don't ever put that in your mind. Just put in your mind that that bitch cancer came in and put your mind in a much better perspective and outlook on life.

I am not saying cancer is a good or easy thing to go through, but if "it" is at your front door don't be afraid or get scared. It, cancer just might be there to empower you, or just simply be there to prove to you that you are a much stronger person than you ever thought. Either way, take what you get out of it and that will be your answer when you ask God why you.

AFTER

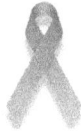

After your treatment finishes eat, eat, eat everything so you can to gain your weight back as fast as you can. If you only gain a little weight, that's ok, so be it. Don't ever wear those hideous cancer wigs. They have some very good lace front wigs you can use, if you're inclined. If you're a white lady don't feel embarrassed to put on a lacefront wig. It will look much better than those horrible looking cancer wigs. Just go to the 'hood to get it done. They do the best job when applying lace front wigs. Don't be scared to go to the hood, the hood doesn't bite. This is the time you need to step outside your box. Just remember, it's a new you because the sooner you start looking good and feeling good, the sooner you'll feel your life go back to normal.

I started feeling good right away, not even a day later, because somehow, I stumbled on a girl on the internet. I don't know how I did that because I don't like the internet. Her name was Lizzo. Her music took me over, and I got hooked. I listened to her music the rest of that year. Her music put my mind in a place as if I never had cancer.

There was another girl, her name was Sharleen. She was so funny. She dresses like an old church lady, and the things she does when imitating them is hilarious. She had me laughing so hard she left me with no cancer in mind.

Then a girl named Nicole. Now she is just plain dumb lol to say the least. She wasn't dumb as being stupid dumb, it was like a funny dumb. The first video I saw of her she was with a damn curling iron, trying to straighten her hair—had me rolling. From there I watched all of her videos. Even to this day I still watch those three girls. Little do they know they helped a cancer ridden man get back to normal, faster than most.

This is where you start to put in your mind that that bitch cancer never happened. When you do this, it makes what you just went through a thing of the past much faster. For me I just put the thoughts of cancer in the most tiniest of places in my mind, so that it never comes out to bring any memories. This is why I made the decision early on only to tell the people in my close circle about me having cancer. I knew they would know how to respect my decision of not speaking of me going through cancer, ever again.

As I am coming to the end of writing this book a pandemic has broken out. The whole world went crazy with everyone having to wear masks when leaving their homes. People with underlying medical conditions were told to stay home, in fear that we may be more at risk. For me, they weren't talking about ME staying at home, because that would make me go crazy. I took all the necessary precautions and went on about my way, because even though I was certain about my mind set about cancer, this was something different, something that no doctors had ever seen before. So yeah, it gave me concern. I was never worried, because if I caught it, I would fight like hell to stay alive, but still I was cautious, after all it's something I didn't want to come my way.

During this time my grandmother who I

spoke of in the beginning, passed away in October 2020. I was advised by my doctor to not travel. Me being who I am, with fear in mind, was not going to let any doctor tell me not to attend my grandmother's funeral in Jamaica.

We had been on lock down for so long, I really needed to get away or I would have gone mad. So, I went and got my Covid-19 test, got on the plane to Jamaica to see my grandma for the last time, came back home, and took another Covid-19 test. The funny thing is while I visited my grandmother's house, and visited family, there was no case of coronavirus in her community. It was more detrimental to my health to be in America, because the virus was claiming more lives in America than anywhere else in the world.

When I got back home, I found out that a very close friend of the family found out she had cancer. She is going through cancer treatment as I'm writing this book. It took me a while to reach out to her because I didn't want her to feel as if she was sick or ill. So I waited and waited till one day I called and told her that I had something for her. It was a flower vase that I had made for her. I didn't want to talk to her as if I needed to know what she was going through. I just wanted it to be like a normal visit where she talked and I listened, because what most people don't understand is that in her situation she didn't need the extra questions, the extra concerns. She just wants you to listen and talk about other things. She didn't need to be reminded about what she was going through. She already knew what she was going through, so I talked to her about what's going on in the world, like the pandemic, life, kids, the usual.

Then I told her before I left, "You got this." I told her how strong people in our culture are and how we've been through the struggles of not having, the hunger of not eating, and the pains of uncertainty. In our minds if we can rise from all of that, then we can rise from anything that comes our way. Our minds are trained and programmed so that anything we face in life we will fight to overcome. We do this as long as we have breath in our body. This has been the mindset of the poor people living in Jamaica for generations.

I told her that I am here if she needs anything, for her to just reach out. However for some strange reason I felt weird telling her about my own personal experience in fear that she might tell others. I still don't want anyone to put my name and cancer in the universe. In my mind, I don't want that dark cloud hovering over my head. It was weighing on my mind to have a talk with her, to pour some of me, my strength, and my positive mindset into her thinking. I thought that maybe something I might say may uplift her on one of her down days, or maybe something I might say may just give her the extra strength to get up, get out, and fight!

I truly believe it was the way I set my mind at the beginning, that helped me go through this process with such ease, more than others. It is also because I always kept a positive attitude. I never complained, never dwelled on what was happening day to day. I just showed up, did what I had to do and never spoke of it.

To this day I never spoke of it, even when it was done. That's where I left it, at the cancer center where it belongs. Because of how my mindset was at that time, my doctors asked me if I wanted to come back and sit with people that were going through cancer treatment, or just to be with them when they were going to listen to how their treatment plan will be. The doctors told me they have never see seen anyone go through the whole nasopharyngeal treatment without having any symptoms. They asked me how I did it.

I wrote this book detailing what I did, hoping it will help as many people as possible. This way if and when they hear the word cancer for the first time it can help them get their mind ready for what's to come. If those words don't give you strength, and the willingness to fight, then remember the good times in your life and rely on them. If all that doesn't work then maybe this will.

There was another person at the treatment centers that amazed me and the doctors. She was a 70-year-old lady. I was told she caught the bus to and from the treatment center. This references the poor people problem I wrote about earlier, and she did all this during winter time. She also had a positive attitude and outlook. Just to know that she had to take the bus in the dead of winter with no complaints, and came in everyday with a positive attitude, taught me the value of strength. She showed me, if she can do all that back and forth, maintain the schedule in and out of the treatment centers, and still have the strength to show and have a positive attitude then I can certainly go through my treatment with ease.

If my words didn't help on any particular day, I would think about that 70 year old lady on the bus. That thought would give me the extra boost to keep fighting while having a positive outlook and attitude. I was so glad the staff told me about her, but for some reason I never got a chance to meet her because our treatment schedules were not the same. When I was finished with my treatment, I was out of there because I felt like if I stuck around, somehow cancer might become my reality. I was set on not making cancer a reality of mine. It will always remain as something I just needed to do at that moment and that's it.

I found out that another person I know has cancer. I felt somewhat hesitant in sharing my experience with her. In a way, I felt guilty. I felt that if I can at least share some of what I went through with her, and how I dealt with it, maybe somehow it could put her mind in extra fighting mode.

I realize that it's just my fear of telling

someone outside my closest family that somehow my cancer experience will always linger out there, and I don't want that. It's my way of saying that I don't want the universe having the knowledge of that kind of disaster, with my name attached to it.

My theory of cancer is even though the doctor said I am free of cancer, when that time comes I know that this is not so. I know that dirty bitch is laying somewhere inside me waiting, but I will also be waiting to kick it's ass again. If I was cancer, I would stay way, way away from me, because this man is a beast.

I know one must be wondering why I call cancer a bitch? When we had very bad storm in my country they would say mother earth is upset, so I figure cancer just might be a mother earth kind of cell going after all the good cells. If cancer is a pissed off mother earth cell bringing the wrath, then why is it name cancer (Can, Sir) and not Canmom (Can, Mom.)?

I hope that reading this book can give a sense of my personality, mindset, fight and how I dealt with such an ordeal. Yes, it's not an easy cake walk, but I truly believe if you have the right mindset and personality, it can truly help you especially on the days when you're feeling down. What I've written in this book helped me, so I am hoping it will help you too.

When I completed my last dose of radiation therapy, everyone including my doctor was amazed that I did all my treatments yet I showed no sign of weight loss or hair loss. I had none of the symptoms or side effects that were expected. My personality and attitude stayed the same. This is why I was asked by my radiation doctor if I would like to come back to the Pet Center (radiation department) to talk to new cancer patients.

I told him no, because being the person I am, I wanted to put the word cancer in the smallest box in my mind and leave it there, never to be reopened or spoken of ever again. This is why I choose to write this book. I figured this is a great way of making myself available, and willing to talk to new cancer patients. This is my way of helping them to get their minds the way mine was at the beginning and end of my cancer treatment.

I hope as you read this book, you will get your mind in the right frame of mind, which is to **FIGHT**. Make your own **HAPPI-NESS**. **CRY** only once, if need be, but please no more than three days. Let the sad time be over. **DON'T TELL THE WORLD**. Only tell the ones closest to you. Try to replace everything that radiation and chemo will destroy in your body, and don't forget that it's ok if you stand in front the mirror everyday throughout whatever treatment plan you have and say, "BITCH YOU CAME FOR ME, BUT FUCK YOU."

Remember by doing so, you're telling cancer it's time to go to war, and you're not ready to back down. If anyone brings that word CANCER up to you during this time, just simply look at them and say, "**FUCK CANCER** . "